DIY Pain Relief

Self Massage and Stretching for Relief of Muscle Pain

© Wesley R. Chaplin

Chapter 1 Muscle Pain and You … 5

Pain and DIY Relief

Tools of the Trade

Chapter 2 The Neck … 13

Introduction to Neck Pain

Neck Anatomy

Neck Pain Relief

Chapter 3 The Upper Body … 23

Introduction to Shoulder Pain

Upper Body Anatomy

Shoulder and Upper Back Pain Relief

Chapter 4 The Low Back … 35

Introduction to Low Back Pain

Lower Back Anatomy

Lower Back Pain Relief

Chapter 5 The Upper Legs ... 47

Introduction to Hip and Thigh Pain

Upper Leg Anatomy

Hip and Leg Pain Relief

Chapter 6 The Lower Legs ... 59

Introduction to Calf and Shin Pain

Lower Leg Anatomy

Pain Relief

Chapter 7 The Feet ... 67

Introduction to Foot Pain

Foot Anatomy

Pain Relief

About the Author ... 76

Chapter 1
Muscle Pain and You

Section 1
Pain and DIY Relief

As a Licensed Massage Therapist, daily I see clients that suffer from muscle tightness, soreness, fatigue, and chronic pain related to muscular issues. Many of these issues can be relieved or prevented with proper stretching and self-massage. Even in cases that are not solely muscular, often there is much that can be done to relieve some of the pain. DIY Pain Relief aims to help give understanding of muscular pain and techniques that an individual can do to help relieve some of that pain.

The most common areas that I see muscle pain that can be avoided or gain relief from self-help are:

Neck and Shoulders A common place that many people hold their stress and a result of bad posture.

Lower Back and Hips Both common issues because they are used constantly and suffer greatly from bad posture, often from long periods of time sitting.

Legs Commonly seen in athletes and active people, but also prevalent in people that stand for long periods of time.

Feet One of the most frequent areas that people have muscular issues and don't realize it. Improper footwear contributes greatly to common foot issues.

As stated before, the two most effective ways to help relieve pain that an individual can do, is to stretch that muscle and the muscles related to or connected to it, or to self-massage the corresponding muscles using the hands or tools (homemade or store bought). These two techniques can be used separately or together to relieve tight muscles and get rid of painful knots.

Massage causes physiological changes to the body through the use of mechanical responses. The mechanical responses are physical effects that occur in the body in response to pressure being applied to the soft (muscle) tissues.

Taking advantage of a little knowledge, anyone can use similar techniques to help elicit mechanical responses in their own muscles with stretching and self-massage techniques.

Stretches can be one of the best ways to actual help relieve muscle pain. Stretching helps create a mechanical response in the muscles to relax and release tension. With a little understanding of the muscles and specific stretching techniques used to isolate the sore muscle, many pains can be worked out. Stretching is an effective technique for relieving muscle pain caused when muscles are tight or cramping.

If your muscles are sore from working out, they are often sore from being used or torn and lengthened. For

6

this reason, pain relief through stretching is not normally affective or highly beneficial for weakened muscles that are already lengthened or overstretched.

Proper form and technique are important when stretching, if the body is in the wrong position, even slightly, depending on the area, can cause strain on a different muscle or the one you are trying to stretch. Proper form is also important to prevent the pinching of any nerves or aggravating the skeletal system.

There are also many tools that can be used to force a stretch, these tools may or may not be harmful and easily misused, for this reason we do not recommend the use of any stretching machines. Any part of the body can and should be stretched with your own weight, control and strength. However, there are some useful tools that can be used to aid in stretching. The easiest and most common is a length of fabric like a towel or even a rope. A towel can help you to reach areas that you might not be able to reach on your own - such as your toes.

Aside from stretching, self-massage can be beneficial in working out difficult knots in muscles throughout the body. Self-massage involves using your hands or tools to apply pressure to muscles in the same way as applied by professional massage therapists. By using these tools, you can often relieve a variety of muscle pain by working out knots or relieving tightness. Self-massage techniques can also be used with stretches to help get into deeper muscles or apply greater pressure to sore areas. This common technique used by massage therapists is known as "pin and stretch," and is normally done by applying pressure (pinning the muscle) to one part of the muscle and then stretching against that "pinned" point. To get into hard to reach areas for self-massage, it often requires the use of tools that can be bought or easily self-made.

Tools of the Trade

When attempting self-massage, without going and seeing a professional, there are a few essentials tools. While there are dozens if not hundreds of tools and gadgets to choose from online and in stores, there are three most common types that can collectively handle almost any muscles.

The three tools that are needed to achieve the few key techniques that can be used are as follows:

1. The first type is a long thick **cylinder.**

These are normally used to roll along long muscles in the body while applying pressure. These are most commonly seen used for the legs along the outside edge of the thigh.

The foam roller is the best bet and are easy to find cheaply.

DIY (Do-It-Yourself) versions include using bottles or cans but be careful to not use anything glass, which has a risk of breaking. Freezing a plastic bottle of water for small areas is a perfect example of a homemade tool.

These tools and techniques give relief over a broad area and not normally specific points of pain or tension.

2. Second type is a **ball**

A ball is used to get direct and pointed pressure on those hard to reach spots, like the back.

The best bet here is to find a solid ball that is comfortable for you and no need to buy a "special" product.

A **DIY** choice is normally a tennis ball, but any size can work and may work better for specific area (others: golf ball, racquet ball, baseball, etc.)

Two balls can be put together in a sock to allow for massaging multiple points on the body. These are good for hitting both side of the spine when experience back pain. Simply take two balls of the same size and place them in a sock (preferably a tube sock.) Then tie off the end of the sock so the tennis balls stay together.

3. The third type is your **fingers**

Your hands and fingers can be used on those spots that are easy to access while staying relaxed. Manual stimulation can also be replaced by using a stick of some sort instead of the fingers. If your hands or fingers grow tired you should stop.

Some impromptu tools to help apply pressure to specific points can be anything that can be held securely and able to apply deep pressure directly without risk of breaking.

Other common treatments in pain relief include:

- **Apply cold** ice packs to lower any inflammation, normally only needed in the first day of injury. Should be done in intervals no less than 30 minutes apart.

- **Apply heat** to help increase circulation and blood flow to the area stimulating healing.

- **Topical creams** Products such as Tiger balm, Icy hot, or Bio freeze can all be used to help aid in the relief and repair of sore muscles.

Chapter 2
The Neck

Introduction to Neck Pain

The neck is a complicated part of the body which houses critical organs, such as nerves and arteries, while also having an amazing amount of versatility in intricate movements. These abilities are some of the reasons why it can be easily susceptible to injury. The neck can twist or rotate to each side, tilt sideways, upward and downward, while also being able to move in circular motions. On top of all these complicated movements the neck is also connected to the shoulders, sharing several muscles. Neck pain is often associated with or accompanied by shoulder or upper back problems.

Common Problems and Causes

Neck pain can arise is several forms, such as:

- A stiff neck resulting from tight neck muscles

- Headaches and migraines from tight neck muscles connecting to the head

- Pain or difficulty in rotating the head

Often these pains are felt in relation to shoulder and

upper back pains. For more information on how to work with those muscles please consult the next chapter on Shoulder & Upper Back Pain.

Common causes of neck pain in daily life include:
- Bad Posture, such as looking down at phone or book for prolonged time, or holding a phone between your head and shoulder.

- Poor sleeping position, pillows at an uncomfortable height can strain the neck.

- Imbalance in carrying heavy objects on one side of the body, like groceries.

More severe problems often occur when the neck makes a sharp or unexpected movement, such as whiplash or falling on the head.

Cautions:

There are several ways you can help fix and relieve neck pain yourself, but due to the delicate nature of the neck and its complexities it can be risky to work on your own neck if the problem is something deeper than tight superficial muscles. Since the neck is such an important and intricate area of the body it is important to see a physician if you feel any shooting pain, severe or recurring problems. A licensed professional can help determine which self help tools are safe and best to use in providing pain relief.

Neck Anatomy

There are several muscles in the neck, as well as many ligaments and bones, a few key prominent muscles can be easily treated on your own. These major muscles are commonly related to ailments in neck pain. These muscles include the sternocleidomastoid (SCM) and the scalenes in the front and side of the neck, with the traps and levator scapulae being the prominent muscles in the back of the neck.

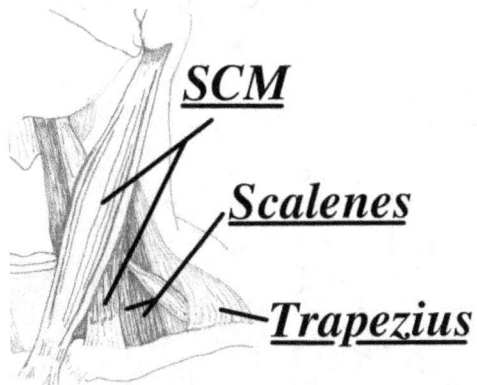

The **SCM** stands for the **SternoCleidoMastoid** which attaches from just below the ear down to the sternum at the top center of the chest. This muscle is often very visible and noticeable on each side of the neck, because the SCM is one of the larger muscles and close to the surface of the skin. The SCM is responsible for rotating the head.

From the front view, it can be seen that there are several smaller muscles behind the SCM. Many of these muscles are the **scalenes**, which connect at the spine in the neck down to the upper ribs. The scalenes help in moving the head laterally and in breathing.

The **trapezius** (shortened to just traps), is a muscle on the back side of the neck that connects to the neck, shoulders and down the length of the upper back. The traps help to connect the shoulder, spine and neck for many complicated movements. Usually the main part of the trapezius that causes neck pain is in the upper portion of the muscle situated in the neck or upper shoulders.

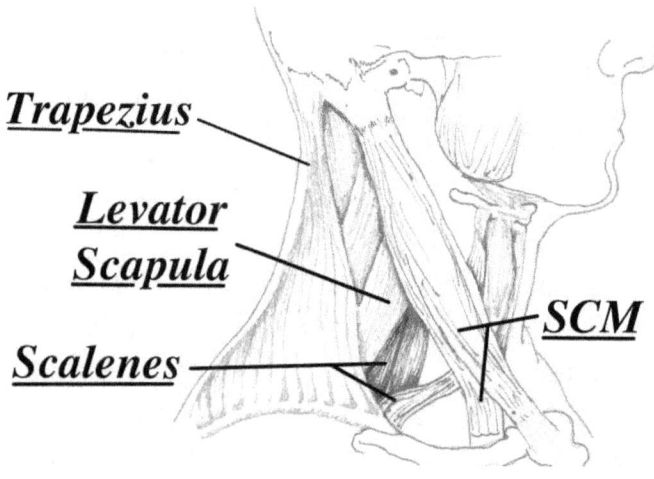

Tension and tightness in the upper traps can put strain on many of the other neck muscles that are not as large or strong, for this reason it is important to look at the Trapezius when trying to determine the source of pain in your neck. Luckily the trapezius is also one of the easiest factors in neck pain that can easily be stretched or self massaged.

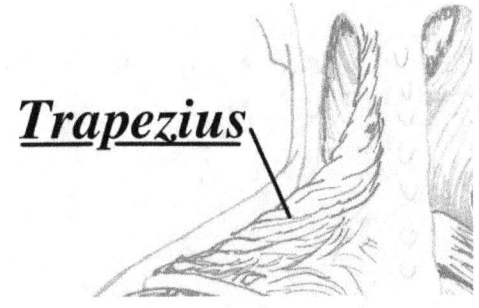

Trapezius

Neck Pain Relief

The key muscles causing many cases of neck stiffness and soreness are large enough for you to be able to use a variety of techniques to relieve the pain.

If you are feeling pain in the back of the neck it is possible to release tension and massage the upper part of the trapezius muscles while also applying deeper pressure into the levator scapulae.

This area is easy to affect through **manual** pressure using the fingers or knuckles

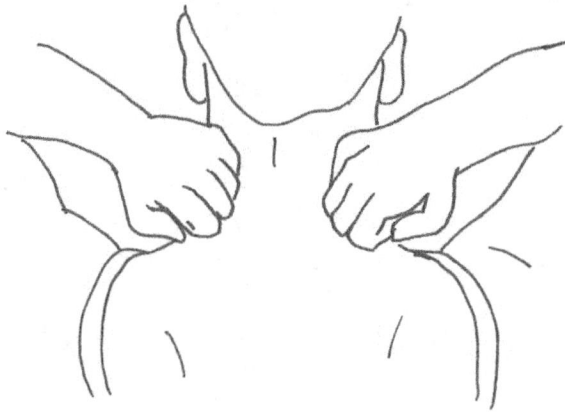

Using you knuckles press into the muscle at the back of your neck along both sides of the spine. Press and hold on areas of tension for 10 - 15 seconds.

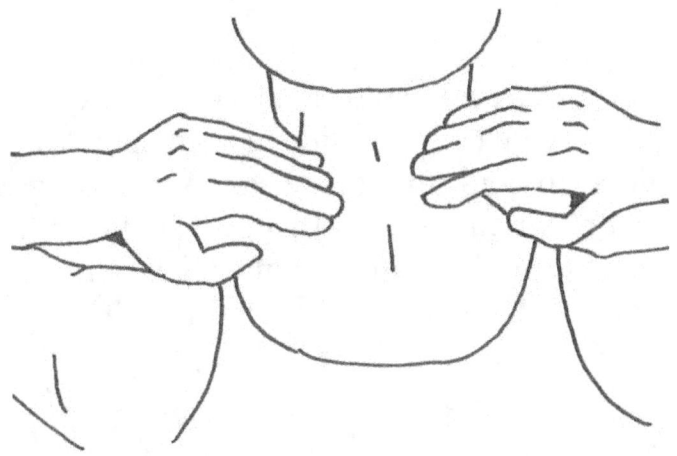

You can also use your fingers instead of you knuckles, this can allow to better grip and slide slowly across any sore areas.

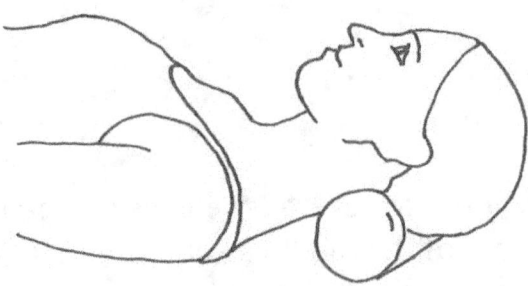

These muscles can also be massaged with a foam **roller** placed under the nook of your neck and rolled back and forth.

Additionally, this area can be reached with the use of a tennis **ball** placed along the side of your spine (this can also be done on both sides at the same time using two balls with or without the sock!). The ball allows for deeper access and the ability to hit trigger points or "knots".)

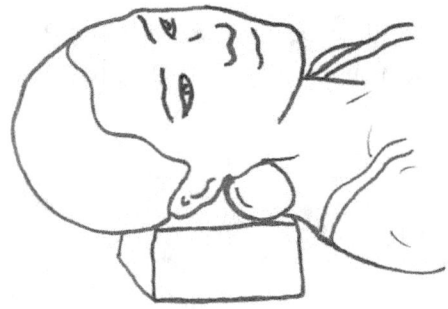

There are also several stretches that can be done to relieve some of the tightness or stiffness in the neck. These stretches can and should be practiced when your neck is not injured. These stretches can help prevent future injuries and increase your neck flexibility.

While standing straight, tilt your head upward as if looking up at the sky directly above you. Isolate your movement to your neck only and keep the rest of your body straight. This helps to stretch and lengthen the SCM and scalenes while contracting and shortening the muscles in the back of the neck (levator scapulae, and others).

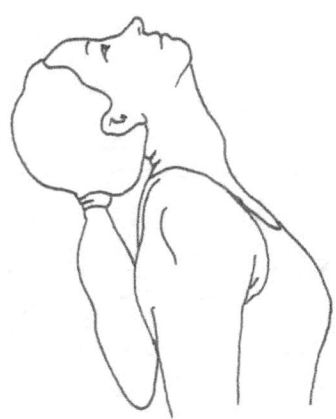

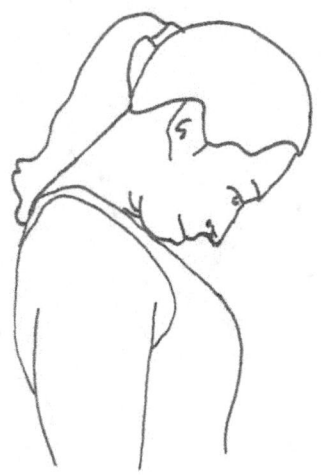

While keeping a straight back tilt your head downward as if looking at your toes. This relaxes the SCM and scalenes while stretching the traps and levator scapulae.

Both stretches can be aided by the hands to get a deeper stretch if desired.

Tilt your head to one side without rotating it. The hand from the same side can help pull the head to the side for a deeper stretch, but it is important to remember to keep your back straight and not to lean or curve your spine to the side. Complete on both the left and right sides.

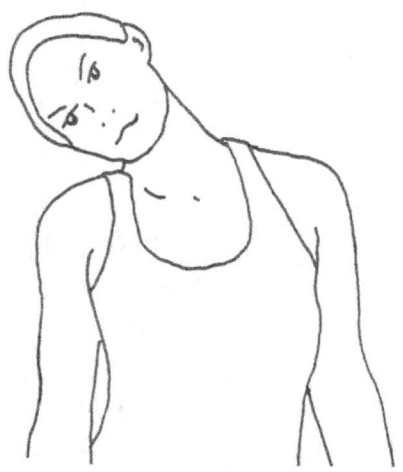

Chapter 3
Upper Body

Section 1
Introduction to Shoulder Pain

Shoulder and upper back pain is extremely common, with estimates of up to 70% of people being affected over the course of their life. The strength and flexibility to reach, hold, lift, carry, press, and pull on a daily basis puts this area under constant stress.

Virtually all our upper body muscles converge with the shoulder in some way and their interrelationship is key for optimal shoulder health and performance. We simply use our upper extremities so much that issues are bound to happen.

Discomfort, if left untreated, can turn into a chronic problem that affects daily activities, such as carrying your groceries and reaching to put them away.

Common Problems and Causes

Shoulder pain is so common because the joint is so frequently used. Any activity that incorporates repetitive movements are capable of causing injury through excessive use, such as:

- Household activities that involve excessive, repetitive arm motion, such as gardening, sweeping, etc.
- Sports that involve that same repetitive arm motion such as tennis, swimming, golfing, etc.

Bad Posture: In this modern era the shoulders are often tight in the front and over lengthened in the back. This is the result of common aspects of life in the digital age. Being bent over and using a keyboard or looking down at the cellphone puts the body in a hunched over position, curling or rolling the shoulders forward.

Any of these activities can cause the muscles to become shortened or over lengthened, both of which are precursors for strains and tears in the shoulder. This type of problem can be helped by massaging and relaxing the chest muscles and stretching by rolling the shoulders back, shortening the over lengthened back muscles.

Cautions:

The complexity of the shoulder and upper back extends beyond just the muscle structure involved. The shoulder is also home to a number bones and ligaments allowing for the wide range of movement performed by the shoulders. For this reason, it is important to be sure that pain and soreness in the area is a result of muscular issues and not something more serious.

Upper Body Anatomy

The anatomy of the shoulder includes not only the muscles connecting to the upper back, but also the muscles in the chest, which are antagonists to the back muscles. Together they connect around the shoulders, working in tension against each other. When one is long the other is short. Poor posture and computer work make it much more common to have shortened muscles in the chest (pectoral muscles) and over lengthened back muscles (rhomboids, traps, levator scapulae).

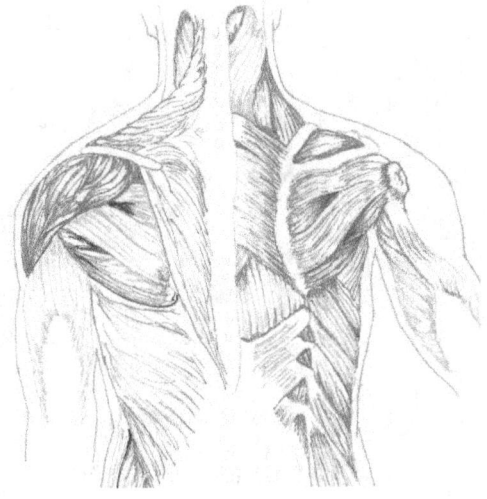

Given that the shoulder contains and incorporates over a dozen different muscles that play a role in the movements of the shoulder, there are several common culprits of pain that can be dealt with on a muscular level.

The major muscles of the **rotator cuff**, which all specifically and primarily deal with the movement of the shoulder are the **Supraspinatus, Infraspinatus, Teres Minor, and Subscapularis** (not pictured). The rotator cuff encompasses the whole shoulder and can be found on top of and above the shoulder blade. The subscapularis is on the inside of the shoulder blade and difficult to get to through self-massage.

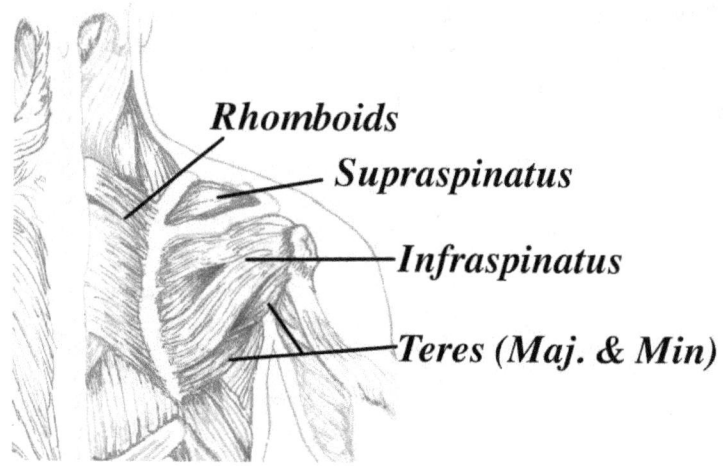

Rhomboids

Supraspinatus

Infraspinatus

Teres (Maj. & Min)

The **rhomboids** rest between the shoulder blades and the spine. These are one of the most common places people have knots in their muscles that cause pain. These muscles help to contract and bring the shoulders back towards the spine. When the shoulders are hunched forward it is the rhomboids that are being overstretched and strained. The rhomboids often pull against the tension of the chest muscles.

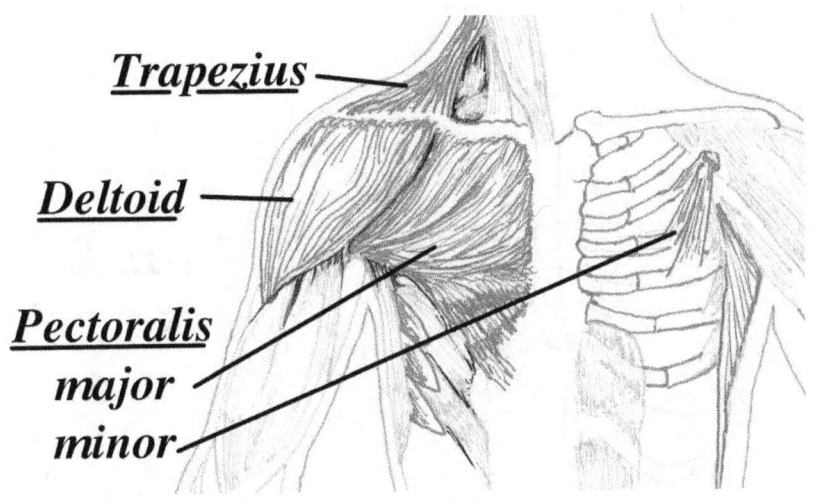

Trapezius ——

Deltoid ——

Pectoralis
major
minor

The chest muscles can also affect the shoulders, especially the **Pectoralis Major** and **Minor** (known as the **Pecs**). The chest muscles, when too tight, pull the shoulders forward and down, stretching against the upper back muscles. Stretching these muscles can help many aches and improve your posture.

One of the largest and most prominent muscles of the shoulder is the **Deltoid** which covers the outside corner of the shoulder. The deltoid plays a role in most shoulder movement and is important in preventing the shoulder from dislocating.

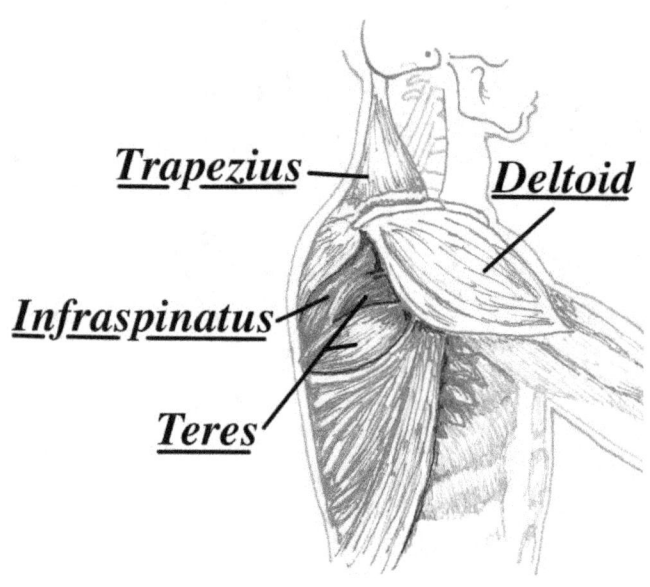

Deltoid injuries are often noted by sharp and severe pain accompanied by swelling. While a deltoid can benefit from massage and stretching, normally if it is sore or injured, it should be examined by a physician to judge the severity of the injury and what exercises are acceptable.

Shoulder and Upper Back Pain Relief

The shoulders often suffer problems from repetitive use. Due to the complexity of the whole shoulder joint, a wide variety of problems can be experienced. Rotator cuff injuries are common, especially if the joint is strained during movement.

Because of the intricate nature of the shoulders and upper back, along with the wide range of areas that can be strained; the techniques listed below are only a few of the many stretches and massage techniques that might be effective. Many of the techniques shown can be applied to the specific area causing pain or related trigger points.

Begin by positioning both hands behind your lower back. Using your right hand grab your left wrist and pull the left arm towards the right side. While gently pulling keep your left arm straight and pointed downward. To increase the stretch in the shoulder and up into the neck the head can also be tilted to the right. This exercise should then be repeated on the opposite side.

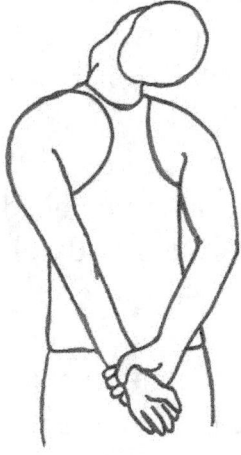

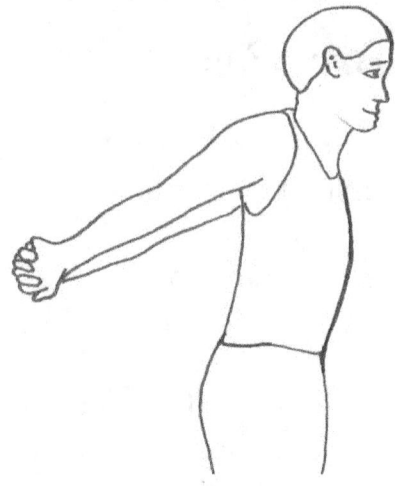

Both arms can also be stretched behind the body. Reach both hands down behind the lower back and clasp them together. Then begin to raise your arms, keeping the hands together. This stretches the chest and rolls the shoulders back.

To help stretch the chest area connecting to the shoulder, you can stretch it along the side of a wall. Standing close to a wall, reach your hand behind you and place the palm of the hand on the wall. Once your hand is placed, you then move your body closer to the wall while keeping the arm straight. The arm can be held at different levels to help fine tune the stretch.

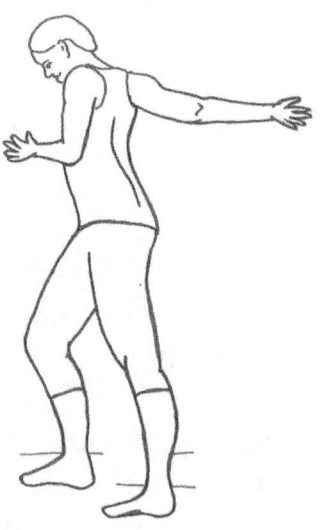

Instead of techniques that always roll the arm behind the lower body it can also be lifted upward. These stretches help to increase flexibility and movement, while also helping to stretch the deltoid muscles as well as the triceps.

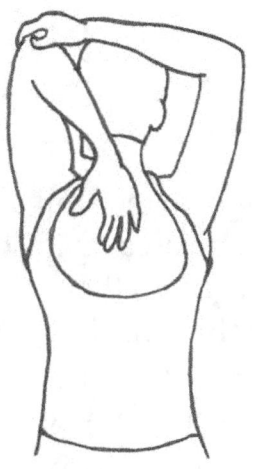

Begin by raising your left arm (bent at the elbow) so that the elbow is pointing upward. The hand and forearm should be bent so that they are facing the upper back (as if you had an itch you were trying to scratch between your shoulders). To aid in the stretch, your right hand can be used to pull the elbow back, deepening the stretch.

If you are not very flexible or are having difficulty with that stretch an alternative version can be done using the aid of a towel.

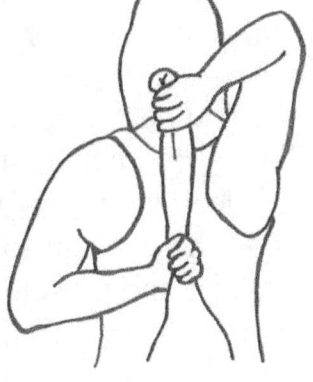

The shoulders and upper back can also be self massaged with the use of a small ball. A smaller ball (at largest the size of a tennis ball) can get into the tight areas and pinpoint areas of pain and trigger points. These self massage techniques can be done against a wall or on the floor.

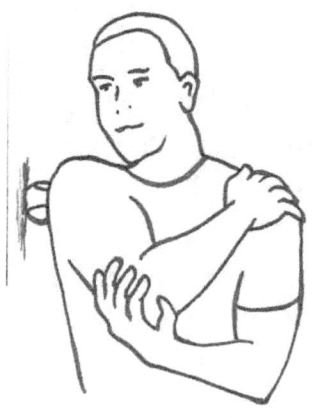

Place a ball against the wall and then lean the sore area against the ball. Leaning into the ball will help it apply specific pressure on the pain area. You can also move your body to allow the ball to roll across a variety of point.

Applying the same technique as with the shoulder, the upper back can also be massaged with a ball. Place a ball against the wall and then lean your back against the ball along the tight muscle. Again, the pressure and muscle being worked can be adjusted by moving; most commonly up and down.

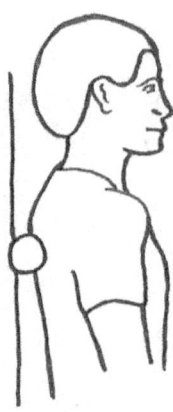

The biggest drawback with these techniques, using a single ball while standing next to a wall, is that the ball can fall loose and drop to the ground. To alleviate this the ball can be placed in a long sock (like a tube sock) and one hand can hold the end of the sock to help keep the ball in place.

An alternative is to do the same self massage techniques while lying on the ground.

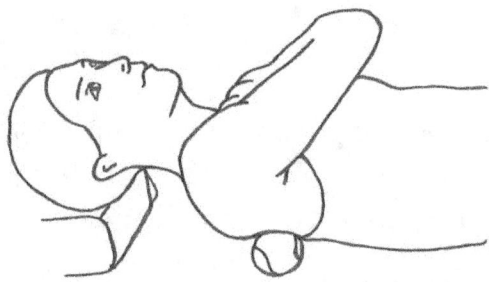

While lying on the ground, lift your shoulder or upper back and place a ball under the sore area. Then relax the body so your own body weight applies the pressure between the muscle and the ball. A block or pillow may be wanted or needed to help keep your head in a comfortable position.

Lying on the ground also allows for the ability to use 2 balls at once, which can be helpful when attempting to massage both sides of the upper back.

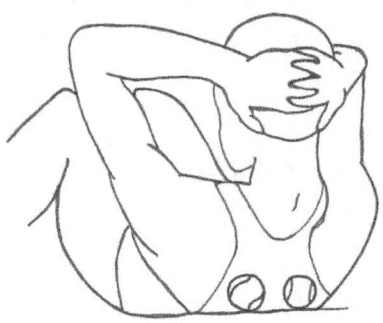

Begin by lying on the ground with your knees bent and your upper back raised. Then place a ball under each shoulder near the spine on opposite sides (you might want or need to place the balls on the ground first.) Then lean your upper back onto the balls, relaxing the weight of your body onto them to a comfortable degree. To work along the spine and the rhomboids you can shift your body weight to roll the balls along these areas.

Chapter 4
The Low Back

Section 1
Introduction to Lower Back Pain

Probably the most common location of the problems I hear about daily is the lower back. Because our backs are used for so much, every activity you perform can put stress on your back. Your back can undergo plenty of strain even during simple, everyday activities such as lifting boxes or walking.

The lower back is under a lot of stress; therefore, it can get fatigued and be a cause of pain or tension in many people. While some of the pains felt in the lower back are from direct issues in that area, many are caused by other muscles attached and near to that area. The lower back is comprised of many muscles connecting the hips to the upper body and lower limbs.

Common Problems and Causes

Depending on the cause, back pain symptoms may be immediately obvious or subtler, manifesting as anything from sharp pain to a dull ache throughout your day. You may find yourself avoiding certain activities that may cause you pain, or pausing often in your routine to try to stretch stiff back muscles. An overstressed back may simply get sore more easily, but a pulled muscle in the back can make it difficult to walk or even move normally at all.

If you have injured your back, you may experience:

- Constant aches or stiffness

- Sharp, sudden pains

- Discomfort and restlessness, or regularly needing to shift position

- Difficulty walking or bending over

Back pain can therefore come from a wide variety of sources, such as:

- Repetitive motion stress from regular physical activity

- Prolonged periods of inactivity, especially from sitting in chairs with poor back support for more than an hour at a time

- Lower back pain may also occur during menstruation

Cautions:

Back pain causes may be as simple as muscle stress, but pain may also be a sign of spinal problems. Be sure to ask a doctor if you think you may have injured your back and are suffering from more than muscle aches. One such common problem is a pinched nerve in the lower back causing shooting pain down the leg, this is known as **sciatica**. Often this pinching is caused by any number of bone and spine issues that are beyond the scope of this book.

Lower Back Anatomy

The lower back and how it connects to the pelvis is complex because it is the main meeting between the torso and the legs. The two large muscles that connect the spine and pelvis are the Quadratus Lumborum (QL for short) and the psoas muscles. The tension and fitness of each one of these muscles can have a large influence on the tilt of the pelvis. The tilt and tension on the pelvis can deeply affect the other muscles connected to the pelvis as well as influence many other body mechanics that can eventually lead to muscular issues in other regions of the body.

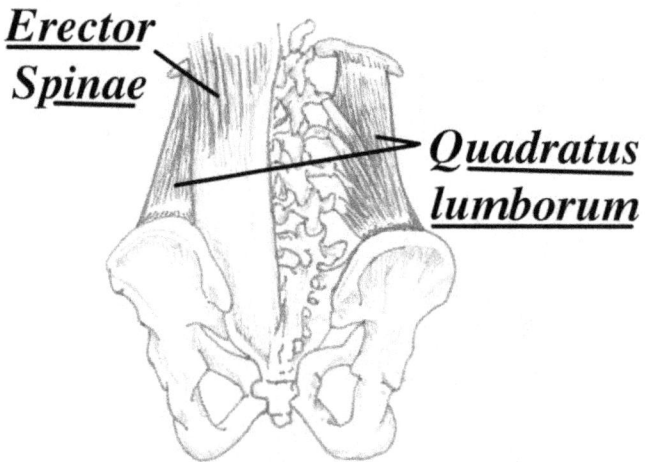

Erector Spinae

Quadratus lumborum

The **erector spinae** are a group of long thin muscles connecting the spine together that run along the entire spine. These groups stretch into the lower back but are normally not the cause of the most common back pain, rather, other surrounding muscles pick up the slack, in turn becoming strained and possibly weakened.

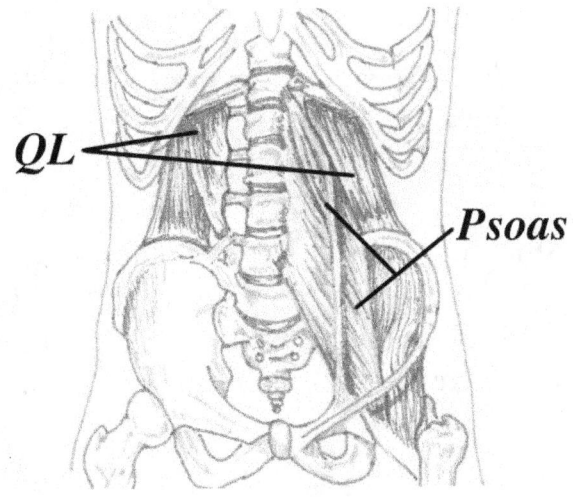

The **Quadratus Lumborum (QL),** is the deepest muscle in the abdomen, but is regularly referred to as a back muscle. It is a broad band that attaches from the lowest rib, or "floating" rib to the top of the iliac crest. It is also more broad on the bottom than on the top. The QL is important due to its pivotal function in normal body mechanics and our upright posture.

The QL can also be weakened or sore due to the **Psoas** muscle being tight. The psoas muscle is also located deep in the abdomen and attaches to the spine. The psoas connects the spine to the lower limbs by connecting to the femur (upper leg). When the psoas is tight it can affect the tilt of the pelvis and tension in the hips, which can cause added strain to the low back and the QL.

Lower Back Pain Relief

One of the easiest ways to gently stretch and relax the back is commonly found in Yoga with a pose called Child's pose. Begin with your hands and knees on the floor, with your knees comfortably apart and the toes touching. Sink your weight back to place your buttocks on your heels. Then reach your hands upward to lengthen and straighten the back before bending forward until your hands are flat on the ground in front of you.

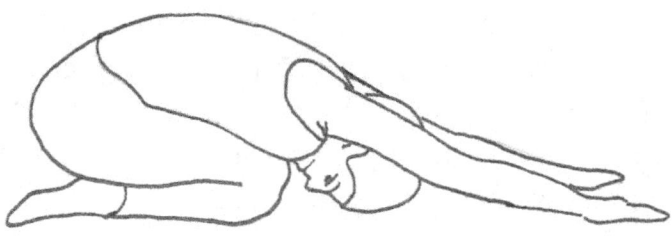

Another common and easy stretch can be done by coming out of Child's pose back up into a position with both hands and knees on the ground with your shoulders above your hands and your hips above your knees.

In this position, flex your back into a rounded position as if pushing your body upward. As your back rises you can also bend your head towards the floor to increase the stretch in the neck and upper back.

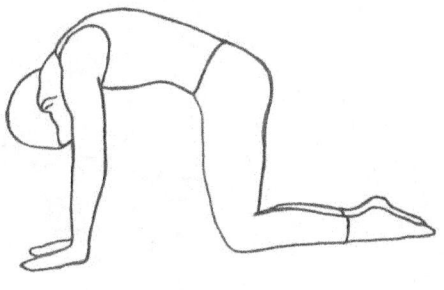

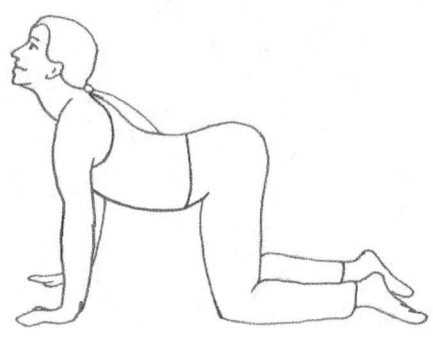

This exercise with the back can also be done in the opposite direction. Still on hands and knees, push your lower back downward towards the ground while lifting your head and upper back upward.

There are also several ways to stretch the lower back from a lying down position as well. Begin by laying flat with your belly on the ground. Support your upper body with your elbows and forearms on the ground. If you are comfortable and desire a deeper stretch you can push your chest upwards.

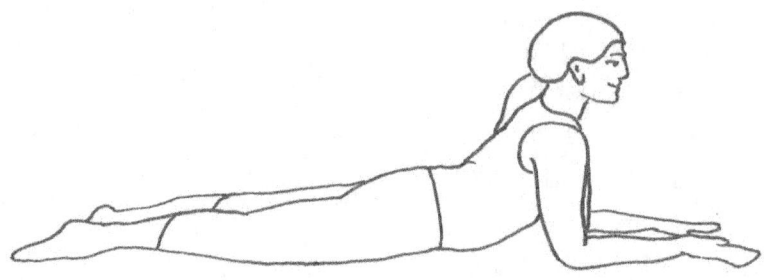

In this elevated position the psoas muscle is being stretched while the lower back muscles can relax. As the psoas loosens it will release tension pulling against the back via the pelvis bone.

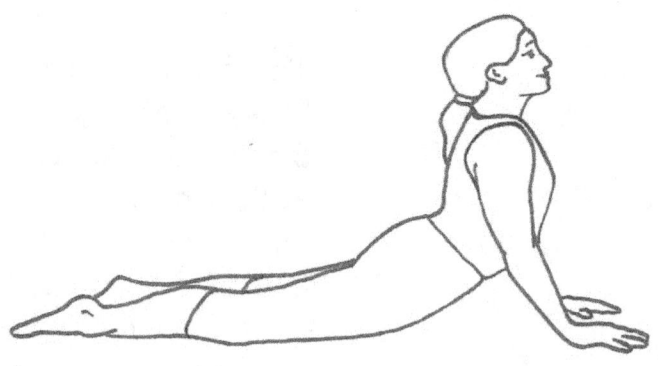

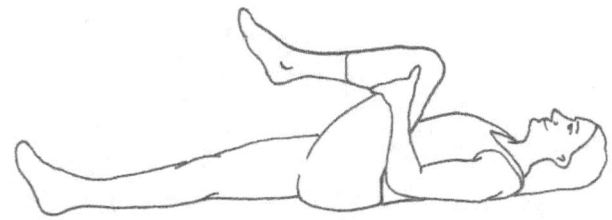

Laying on your back you can also stretch the lower back by lifting one bent leg at a time towards the chest. This stretch isolates one side of the QL muscle at a time. Simply pull one knee straight towards your chest allowing the lower leg to bend and relax.

Another stretch can be done with the leg bent while laying on your back. Take the bent leg and allow it to cross over the other. Keeping your leg bent and the thigh at a 90-degree angle, let your knee drop towards the floor. The pelvis and hips should be twisting to the side as the shoulders remain on the ground. This stretch helps to stretch the QL from a different angle than the previous stretches, as well as stretching the hip muscles and the connection between the lower back and hips.

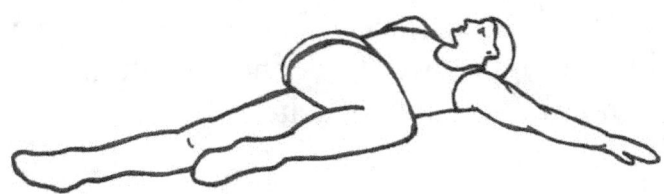

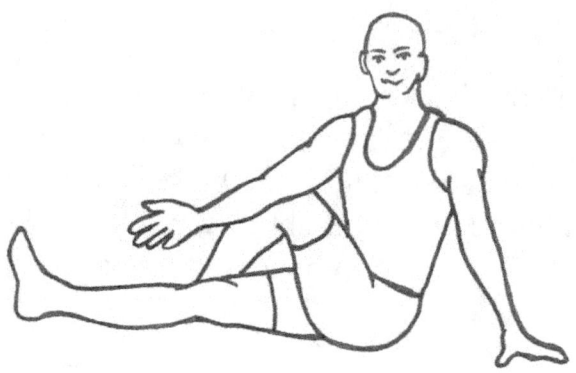

A similar stretch for the low back and hip complex of muscles can be done in a seated position. Begin by sitting on the ground with your legs straight out in front of you. Bend your left leg and place the foot over your right leg placing the foot near the opposite knee. Then rotate your upper body to the left so your right arm is over your left knee while supporting your balance with your left hand. A deeper stretch is achieved by pushing the elbow against the knee to help rotate the torso, stretching the right lower back and the left hip. This can then be practiced on the opposite side.

Foam rollers can also be used to help massage sore muscles in the lower back by sitting in a similar position as to the previous stretch with one leg crossed over the other. Place a foam roller under your hips, just below the lower back, and shift your weight back and forth on it, rolling over your lower back muscles.

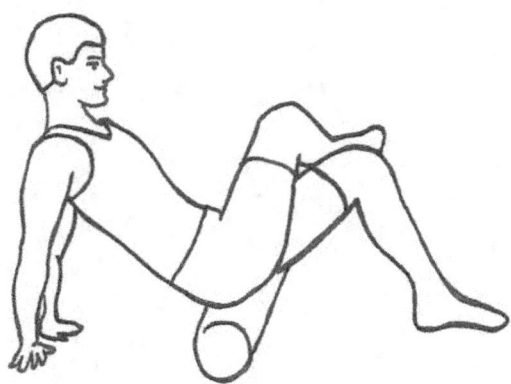

Chapter 5
Upper Legs

Section 1
Introduction to Hip and Thigh Pain

The muscles in the upper leg, including the hip, butt, and thigh, all contribute to common muscle pain felt in the lower body. The quadriceps and hamstrings, balance each other while promoting joint stability and being shock absorbers. The hips and butt muscles help with hip movement and connecting to the upper body.

The most common problems in the leg often relate to the joints of the knee and hip. While these specific problems are a separate issue in and of themselves, the muscles connected to them can exacerbate joint problems. Even if the muscles of the upper leg are not directly feeling pain, it is still important to make sure that they are not tight, which can happen slowly over time, for this reason regular stretching will help prevent injury.

Common Problems and Causes

Upper leg pain symptoms range from those that are hard to detect to those that make you want to stay in bed. Depending on the cause of your upper leg pain, the symptoms may be different.

Upper leg pain symptoms can range from occasional aches and pains, including muscle cramps or sore muscles, including:

- Pain around the front of the thigh, in the quads (Quadriceps)

- Pain in the back of thigh in the hamstrings

- Pain and tightness on the outside of the leg caused by the IT Band and TFL

These pains can be caused by:

- Hamstring injuries

- Overuse of hip - common in runners and athletes

In addition, athletes are also more prone to suffer from upper leg pain in the muscles. Activities such as running, soccer, hiking, etc all involve intense or long periods of time utilizing the upper leg muscles, increasing the likelihood of strain. An overuse injury might begin to ache a little after you participate in an activity but get gradually worse over time.

Overuse injuries can be avoided if you know how to stretch, rest, and perform with proper techniques.

Pulling at the front of the thigh along with a feeling of tightness is a common and minor problem that can be dealt with personally through stretching and self massage. However, if the pain is sharp and acute this could be a more severe muscle sprain or even tear, which should be seen by a professional.

Cautions:
Swelling and stiffness in the joints of the hips and knees are often indicative of a more serious problem that would require medical consultation from a professional.

In addition, **sciatica** is felt as a tingling or numbness down the side of the leg, but, in reality, this is likely caused by a nerve issue stemming from the lower back.

Upper Leg Anatomy

The quadriceps and hamstrings are the two paired muscles of the legs along the front and back side of the upper leg. These muscles work to control the knee and help us bend our leg. When one contracts the other relaxes because they are antagonists.

The **Quadriceps**, or simply **quads**, are four large muscles that make up the front portion of the thigh, which primarily help to extend the knee. These four muscles are the rectus femoris, vastus medialis, vastus lateralis, and the vastus intermedius (not shown). The main muscle that is felt on top of the thigh is the rectus femoris, while the vastus muscles are to the side and behind it. These muscles are often a common point for pain, especially in athletes, because of their use in running. Because of the attachments to the knee, these muscles can exacerbate joint pain if the muscles are tight or sore.

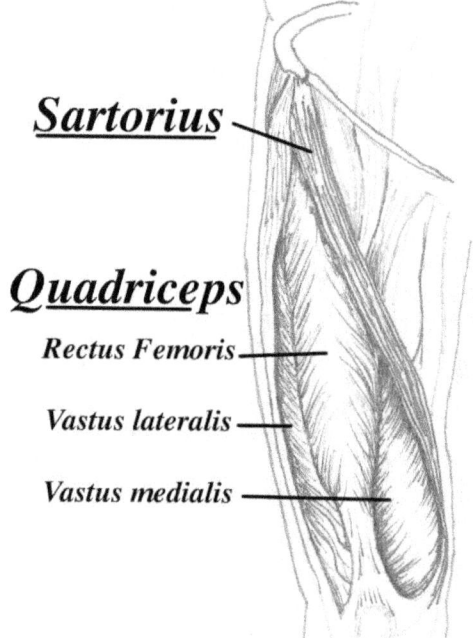

Sartorius

Quadriceps

Rectus Femoris

Vastus lateralis

Vastus medialis

Along the inner thigh, wrapping over the top edge of the quadriceps, is the **Sartorius.** This muscle is a synergist, or cooperative muscle, that is involved in a variety of movements around the hip and knee.

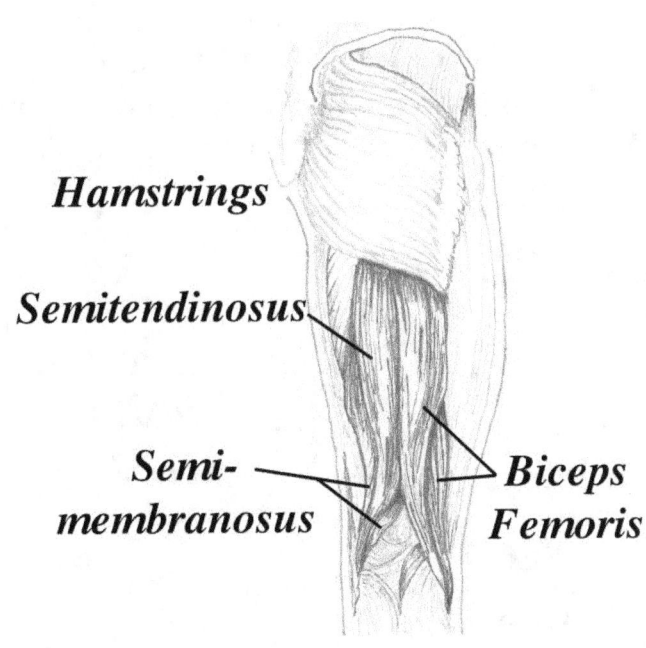

Hamstrings

Semitendinosus

Semi-membranosus

Biceps Femoris

In the back of the legs, acting as an antagonist to the quads, are the **Hamstrings**. The hamstrings are comprised of three muscles: the biceps femoris, semitendinosus, and the semimembranosus. The biceps femoris has two distinct "heads" and in the lower part of the back of the thigh can feel distinctly different. These muscles help connect the pelvis and the knee, helping in the action of flexing and extending the leg and knee.

Along the outside of the leg is a long band of often tight and sensitive fibrous tissue known as the **IT (Iliotibial tract) Band**. This band is an extension of the Tensor Fasciae Latae, also known as the **TFL**. Both the IT Band and the TFL are important muscle structures to know since they can often be related to a variety of hip, leg, and knee pain.

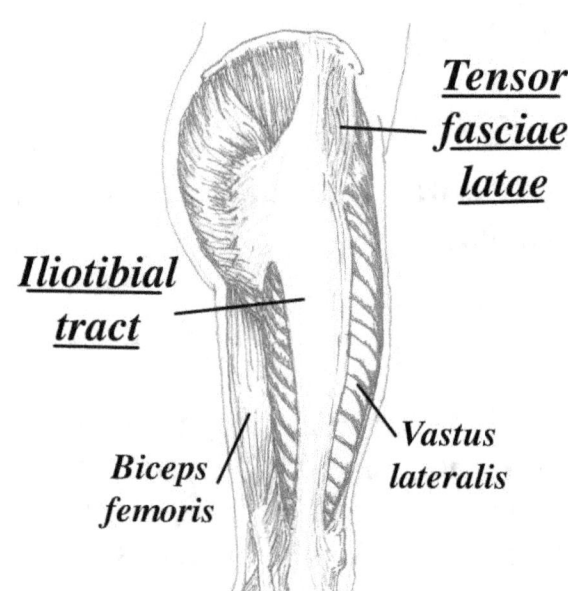

Hip and Leg Pain Relief

You can perform several good upper leg stretches in a standing position. While standing with your right leg slightly bent straighten your left leg out straight in front of you placing your heel on the ground a foot or two in front of you. Leaning forward place your hand on the top of your left thigh. Here pressure can be applied down onto the leg to both deepen the stretch and /or massage the upper leg. The **hamstrings** are stretched and the **quads** are being massaged.

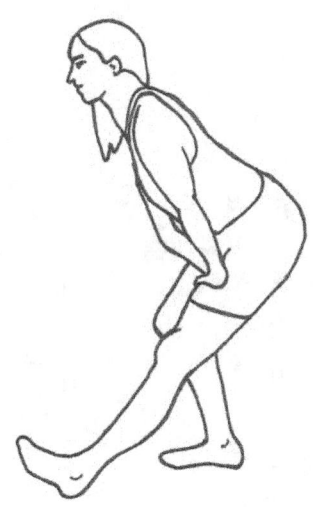

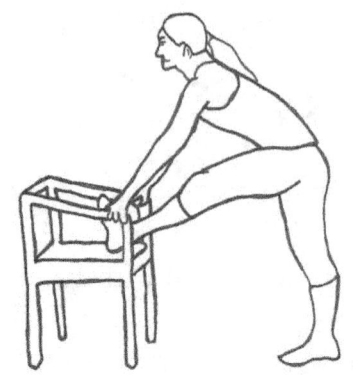

With the aid of a chair this stretch can be enhanced. Begin by placing your left leg on the seat of a chair that is at a comfortable height. Straighten both legs and lean your upper body forward towards the chair. The chair can also be used for balance if it has arms that are within reach. This focuses on stretching the **hamstrings,** but can also help the lower back as well.

A chair can also be used for balance in other standing stretches. The **quads** can be stretched by standing on the right leg while bending your left knee so the foot is behind the buttocks. Use the left hand to grab a hold of the left foot and help press it towards the butt.

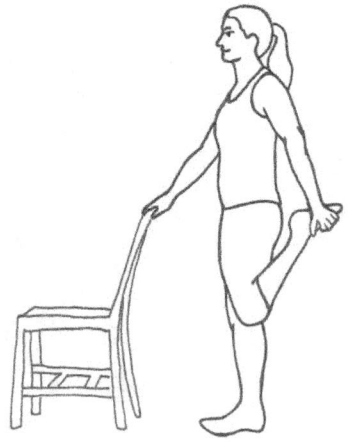

A foam roller can also be a very useful tool in working out tightness in the upper legs and is often seen being used by runners and athletes. Begin in a seated position on the floor with your legs bent, then lift your hips and place a foam roller under your left leg.

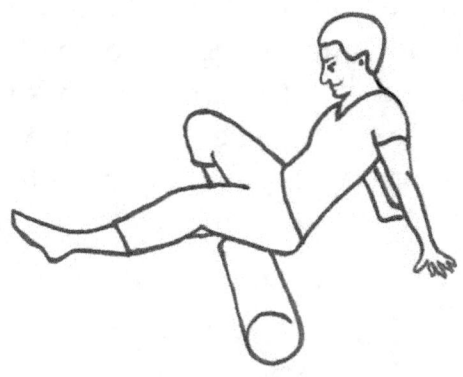

After placing the foam roller under your left leg extend the leg and support your body weight with your hands. Roll your body weight forward and back to help massage the **hamstring** muscles in the back of the leg. Repeat this on the right side as well.

Similarly, the foam roller can be placed on the outside of the legs.

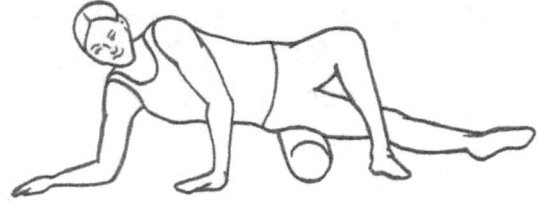

Rotate your body to the side so the body weight is on your right arm and your left leg is crossed over the right leg with the foot on the ground. Then lift your hips and place a foam roller along the outside of the right leg, move back and forth with your body weight to massage the **IT band**.

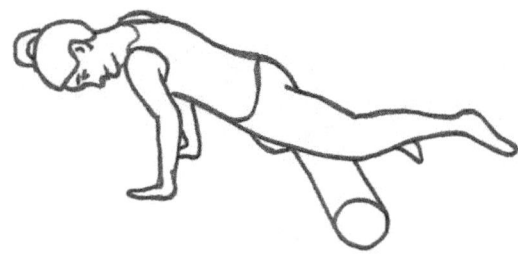

The thigh and quads can also be massaged using a foam roller. Begin by getting in a push up position and then place the foam roller under your left leg. Lower your body weight down so that the right knee touches the ground to help with support and balance, then lower your left thigh onto the roller and shift back and forth across the **quadricep** muscles.

To help stretch the hip muscles begin by lying with your back flat on the ground with your knees bent and feet flat on the ground. Extend your left leg straight in the air so that the bottom of the foot is facing the sky. Then slowly move your left leg directly to the left side. This stretch is a lot easier if you initially do this stretch with the aid of a towel or piece of cloth held at one end in the hand and the other end wrapped around the outside of your left foot. This cloth helps to keep control of the leg and reduce the likelihood of cramping or pinching of your hip muscles.

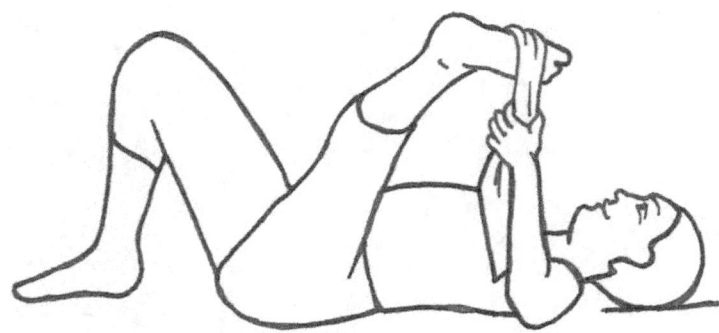

The outside of the hip can be stretched easily in a standing position.

Begin by standing with your left hand against a wall or secure object for balance, then cross your left leg behind your right leg. The left foot should bend so the outside of the foot is on the ground. Slowly bend your supporting leg lowering your body towards the ground while allowing your left leg foot and leg to slide to the right along the floor. As you go lower you should begin to feel a stretch in outside of your left leg. This can be repeated on the opposite side.

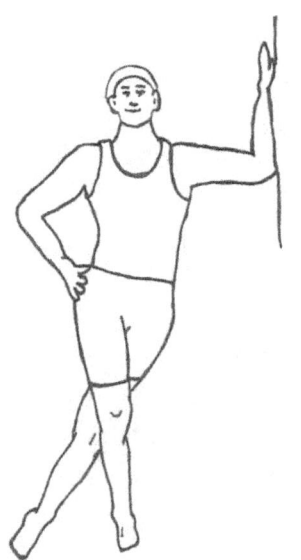
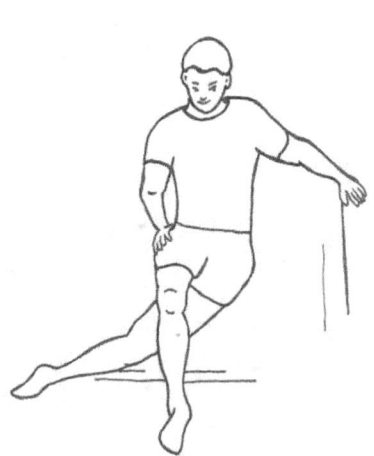

Chapter 6
Lower Legs

Section 1
Introduction to Calf and Shin Pain

The calf is important in walking and connecting to the ankle. The muscles in the front of the leg along the shin help in movement and finer control over the ankle joint. The lower leg takes a lot of pressure everyday because it is used in walking and absorbing the force of the ground. Whether walking, running, or even just standing, the lower leg is always at work. Due to its constant use the calf can be prone to cramps. If this is frequent, drink more water and try some bananas.

The legs may also swell and feel restless especially if much of your day is done standing. If this problem occurs it can be helpful to lay down in a position where you can elevate your legs, such as against a wall. This will help any stagnant blood circulate back towards the torso.

Many lower leg pain causes are due to overuse, sudden change in activity, sports injuries, direct blows to the calf, and not wearing the proper footwear during physical activities.

Common Problems and Causes

Lower leg pain symptoms can range from occasional aches and pains which are often treatable at home, including muscle cramps or sore muscles, causing:

- Pain around the shin bone, commonly called shin splints
- Pain in the calf muscles on the back side of the lower leg.

More severe cases of pain in the lower leg can be causes by inflamed or torn muscles and tendons, causing:

- Tenderness and stiffness, especially in the morning
- Difficulty in going up steps
- Sharp shooting pain in the shins

Be sure to see your doctor if you have any question about your leg pain or if symptoms get worse.

A common problem found in the lower leg can be on the front side most commonly **shin splints**. The muscles on the front of the legs become inflamed making it hard or painful to walk, run, or jump. Commonly caused by doing activity on hard surfaces. Shin Splints can benefit from ice causing the inflammation to go down.

Lower leg pain resulting from muscle issues that can benefit from self massage and stretches are commonly found in the calf. The 2 major muscles that make up the back of the leg can both be easily massaged and stretched.

Lower Leg Anatomy

The back of the lower leg, known as the calf is comprised of two key muscles, the gastrocnemius and the soleus. These muscles are used in walking, hiking, and running, which can lead to sore muscles in the calf. The two muscles in the front of the leg are the tibialis anterior and the peroneus longus.

The back of the calf is covered primarily by a muscle with two distinct halves known as the **gastrocnemius** (or **gastroc** for short) which is connected to the heel by the calcaneal tendon. This muscle and tendon are closest to the surface and take up much of the surface area.

Behind the gastroc is the **soleus** muscle, which is a large muscle that makes up the bulk of the calf. The upper part of the back of the lower leg is covered by the gastroc but as you get lower down the leg, the soleus can be felt directly on the sides of the tendon. The soleus can also be felt on the front of the leg along the inside of the shin.

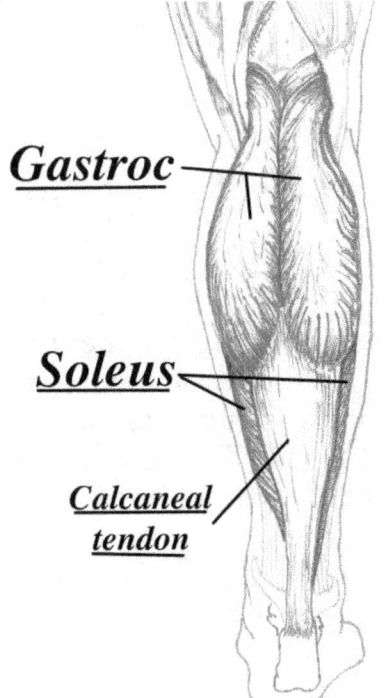

Gastroc

Soleus

Calcaneal tendon

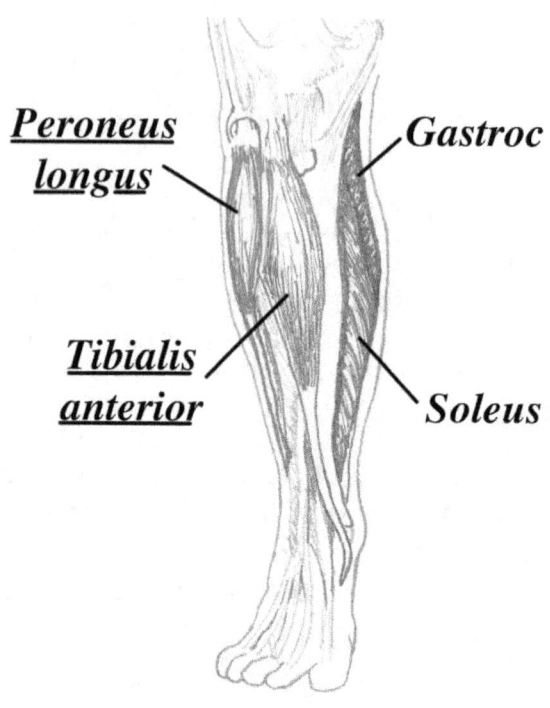

The front of the leg consists of several much smaller muscles. Running along the outside of the leg is the **Peroneus longus** and coming from the knee down along the front to the outside of the shin is the **Tibialis anterior** or simply the tibialis. Both these muscles are used to move the ankle and give it stability. For example, when kicking a ball, these muscles keep your foot "locked" in the desired position. These muscles can be part of the soreness related to shin splint.

Hip and Leg Pain Relief

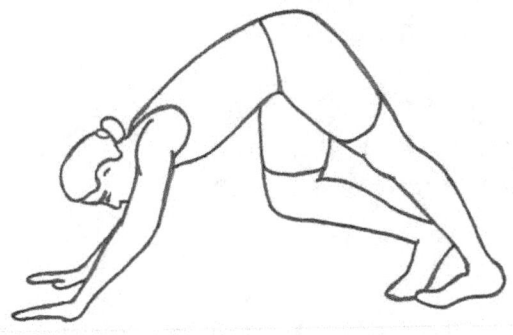

Begin by bending forward so both your hands and the balls of your feet are on the ground. Bend your right leg so that most your weight is on the left foot and hands, then push your weight back into you left heel. This will get a stretch into your **hamstrings,** as well as the calf muscles, the **gastroc** and **soleus.**

A similar stretch can be done standing with the use of a wall. Place both your hands against a wall then step back with your right leg allowing your hips to move back and the left leg to bend. Position yourself as if you are trying to push the wall over. Step far enough back that your right foot is just slightly on the ball of the foot. Then push back into the right heel towards the ground.

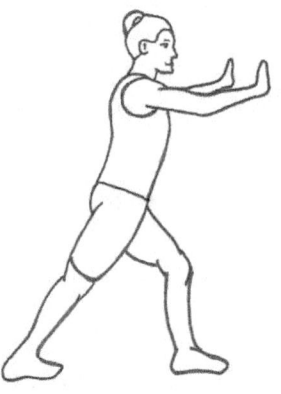

The calves can also be stretched using the edge of a step. Begin by getting in a stable position with your heels facing the edge of the bottom step (don't do this at the top of stairs in case you lose balance.)

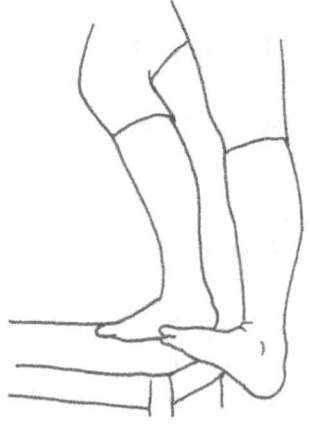

Then take your left foot and place just the toes and ball of the foot on the step, continue by lowering your left heel over the edge of the step stretching the calf muscles. This technique is especially useful if your calf or ankle happens to be more flexible and need a deeper stretch.

While sitting on the floor the calf can be stretched by first sitting on the floor with your right leg extended straight. Then reach forward and bend your toes towards your body. If you cannot comfortably reach your toes then use a length of cloth to help pull the toes and upper foot towards you. This should be done on both legs.

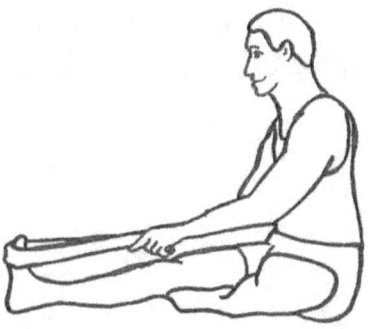

In the same way a foam roller is used to massage the upper legs and hamstrings, it can also be used to massage your calf. Sitting on the ground, support your weight slightly behind you with your hands and place a foam roller beneath your right calf. Then place the left leg on top of your right leg to add more pressure

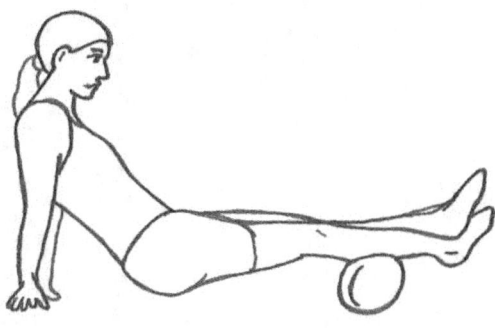

between the foam roller and the sore muscles. Rolling back and forth along the roller to work different points along the calf.

Similarly, this technique can be completed using a small ball in order to get into tighter or more specific points in the calf. The main difference is that you might need to use something to raise the ball to maintain good control and pressure.

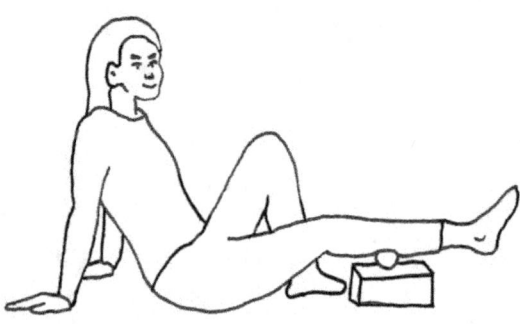

Chapter 7
Feet

Introduction to Foot Pain

The feet are one of the toughest and tense muscles in the body, but because they are constantly being used they are also a common area that can benefit from self massage and stretching. The foot is made up of a complex arrangement of bones, muscles, ligaments and nerves. Problems in any of these structures can lead to pain, weakness, stiffness and abnormal sensations. The type of symptoms, location and severity can help determine what structures are at fault. Other issues such as hammertoes and bunions are not simply muscle issues and a physician should be consulted.

Common Problems and Causes

Foot pain symptoms from muscle problems often present as an achy pain which worsens with activity and eases with rest. Foot pain symptoms vary depending on the underlying problems.

- Pain can also occur simply because of the shape of your foot

- Pain from improper footwear

- Pain underneath the foot or in the foot arch is particularly common in people who spend long periods on their feet.

- Cramping can occur due to mineral and vitamin

imbalance and dehydration

- Plantar fasciitis symptoms of pain and tenderness under the heel are a common problem.

Foot pain can be caused by improperly fitting shoes, so be sure to check your footwear first. The arches of the foot are the primary muscles in the foot that take the brunt of the ground force transmitted into the body.

The arches of the foot are formed by the way the foot bones are supported by various muscles, ligaments and tendons and they control how forces are transmitted through the foot. Pain on the bottom of the foot often results from a problem in the position of the foot arches e.g. having flat feet.

Foot pain symptoms from cramping can be extremely unpleasant, but they are not usually serious. The muscles tighten uncontrollably causing intense pain making it difficult to move. Links have been found between foot cramps and a lack of certain vitamins and minerals, dehydration, lack of exercise, as well as some medical conditions.

Heel pain usually occurs either at the back of the heel or underneath the heel. Our heels absorb most of the force going through our feet so it is a common place to experience foot pain.

Muscle weakness, tightness or overloading often causes pain along the bottom of the foot. They may result in damage to the soft tissues such as plantar fasciitis or tendonitis. Plantar fasciitis is a common cause of heel pain and affects approximately 1-in-10 people. It develops when there is damage and inflammation of the plantar fascia, the thick band of tissue on the sole of your foot. Plantar fasciitis usually develops due to overuse.

The arch of the foot can suffer from tightness and is often the focus of massage techniques to stretch, relax, and relieve pain.

Foot Anatomy

The feet are comprised of many muscles that are thick and tight along the bottom of the foot (the arch). That is why a deep foot massage feels so good.

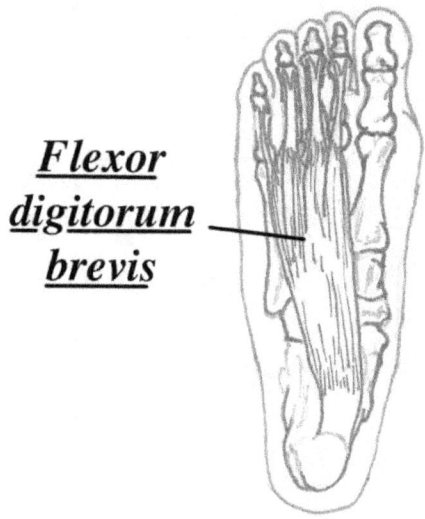

Flexor digitorum brevis

Located in the center of the bottom of the foot is a group of muscles known as the **flexor digitoum brevis**. Think of these as the "arch" of your feet. From a view of the bottom of the foot it can be seen how these muscles attach from the heel of the foot to each of the four smaller toes.

Along the sides on the bottom of the feet there are two muscles, the **abductor digiti minimi and abductor hallucis**. These two muscles help to move the large toe and the little toe on the outer edges of the foot. These muscles are often strained by the shoes we wear, more so than the arch of the foot. Improper shoes can cause the muscles to be in uncomfortable and strained positions for long periods of time, resulting in pain and deformity in the foot.

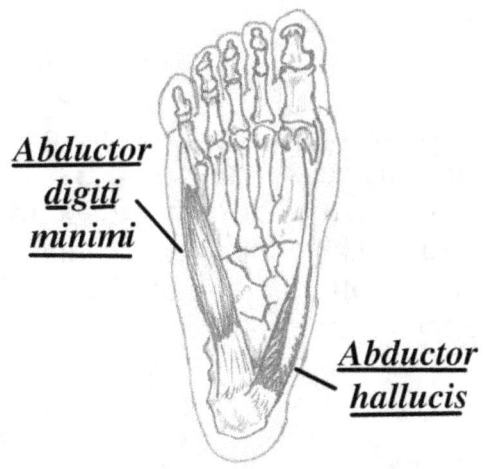

Abductor digiti minimi

Abductor hallucis

On top of these muscles, closer to the surface of the bottom of the foot, is the plantar fascia (not pictured). The **plantar fascia** is a thick, tough, fibrous band made up of collagen fibers, which runs along the sole of your foot. It originates from the heel bone (calcaneus), extends along the bottom of the foot and attaches to the bottom of the toes. It helps to support the arch of your foot and transfers force across your foot when you walk or run.

Foot Pain Relief

Because of the anatomy of the feet, there are only a few ways the actual foot can move (not including ankle movement). The feet can be flexed with toes pointing upward or flexed curling downward. This can be done using the whole foot or isolating muscles related with each individual toe.

While standing, or seated, get in a position where your hand can comfortably reach your foot. Use the palm of your hand to curl your toes downward and towards the bottom of your foot. This helps relieve tension on the taut muscles on the bottom while also stretching muscles on the top of the foot.

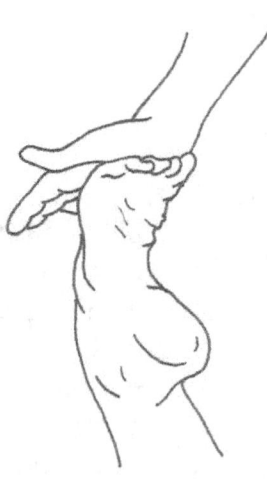

The muscles of the bottom of the feet can be stretched in a similar fashion using the hand to curl the toes upward and stretch the arch of the foot, but due to the thick tight muscles found in the feet this stretch is normally not strong enough. If this is the case, a better technique involves using your body weight to apply the stretch, getting deeper into the arches of the foot.

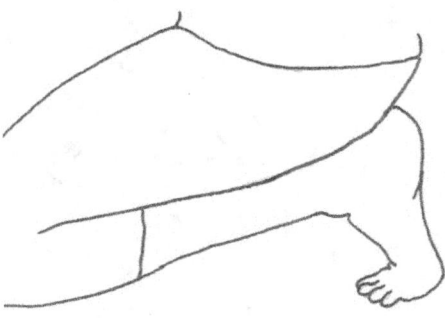

Begin by getting on your hands and knees on the ground, then while slightly shifting your body weight forward lift your feet and curl your toes so they are touching the ground. This arches of the should already be getting a stretch in this position, but it can be made deeper by shifting your weight back until the hips and buttocks touch the heels of your feet.

The feet muscles can also be stretched individually with toe exercises. Sit comfortably with your feet flat on the ground in front of you. Then start by moving and flexing your toes one by one. Each toe will help stretch a different muscle in the arch of the foot. You can also grab each toe and pull it towards you to get a deep stretch if need, but remember individually the toes don't need as much pressure.

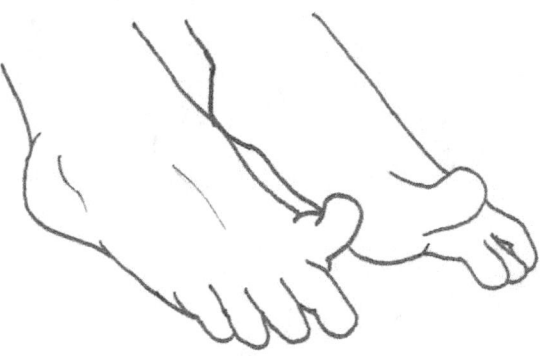

Self massaging the bottom of your foot can be done with either a ball or cylinder shaped object that has some strength. Both are used by placing the ball or cylinder under the arch of the foot then rolling the object along the arch of the foot.

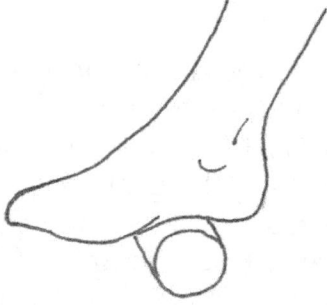

About the Author

Wesley Chaplin is a Licensed Massage Therapist that has been learning and practicing bodywork for 15 years. He has spent over a decade abroad studying and learning traditional massage and stretching techniques in India, China, and Thailand, as well as study of Western Massage in the United States. Today he owns and operates his own massage and wellness studio in Colorado.